RUNNING / JOGGING LOG

YEAR _______ MONTH _______

DATE	DISTANCE	TIME	PACE	HR	REST HR	RUN TYPE	SHOES	NOTES

RUNNING / JOGGING LOG

YEAR _______ MONTH _______

DATE	DISTANCE	TIME	PACE	HR	REST HR	RUN TYPE	SHOES	NOTES

RUNNING / JOGGING LOG

YEAR _________ MONTH _________

DATE	DISTANCE	TIME	PACE	HR	REST HR	RUN TYPE	SHOES	NOTES

RUNNING / JOGGING LOG

YEAR _______ MONTH _______

DATE	DISTANCE	TIME	PACE	HR	REST HR	RUN TYPE	SHOES	NOTES

DATE	DISTANCE	TIME	PACE	HR	REST HR	RUN TYPE	SHOES	NOTES

RUNNING / JOGGING LOG

YEAR _________ MONTH _________

DATE	DISTANCE	TIME	PACE	HR	REST HR	RUN TYPE	SHOES	NOTES

RUNNING / JOGGING LOG

YEAR _______ MONTH _______

DATE	DISTANCE	TIME	PACE	HR	REST HR	RUN TYPE	SHOES	NOTES

RUNNING / JOGGING LOG

YEAR _______ MONTH _______

DATE	DISTANCE	TIME	PACE	HR	REST HR	RUN TYPE	SHOES	NOTES
DATE	DISTANCE	TIME	PACE	HR	REST HR	RUN TYPE	SHOES	NOTES

RUNNING / JOGGING LOG

YEAR _________ MONTH _________

DATE	DISTANCE	TIME	PACE	HR	REST HR	RUN TYPE	SHOES	NOTES
DATE	DISTANCE	TIME	PACE	HR	REST HR	RUN TYPE	SHOES	NOTES

RUNNING / JOGGING LOG

YEAR _______ MONTH _______

DATE	DISTANCE	TIME	PACE	HR	REST HR	RUN TYPE	SHOES	NOTES

RUNNING / JOGGING LOG

YEAR _______ MONTH _______

DATE	DISTANCE	TIME	PACE	HR	REST HR	RUN TYPE	SHOES	NOTES

DATE	DISTANCE	TIME	PACE	HR	REST HR	RUN TYPE	SHOES	NOTES

RUNNING / JOGGING LOG

YEAR ______ MONTH ______

DATE	DISTANCE	TIME	PACE	HR	REST HR	RUN TYPE	SHOES	NOTES

RUNNING / JOGGING LOG

YEAR _______ MONTH _______

DATE	DISTANCE	TIME	PACE	HR	REST HR	RUN TYPE	SHOES	NOTES

RUNNING / JOGGING LOG

YEAR _______ MONTH _______

DATE	DISTANCE	TIME	PACE	HR	REST HR	RUN TYPE	SHOES	NOTES

RUNNING / JOGGING LOG

YEAR _________ MONTH _________

DATE	DISTANCE	TIME	PACE	HR	REST HR	RUN TYPE	SHOES	NOTES
DATE	DISTANCE	TIME	PACE	HR	REST HR	RUN TYPE	SHOES	NOTES

RUNNING / JOGGING LOG

YEAR _______ MONTH _______

DATE	DISTANCE	TIME	PACE	HR	REST HR	RUN TYPE	SHOES	NOTES

RUNNING / JOGGING LOG

YEAR ______ MONTH ______

DATE	DISTANCE	TIME	PACE	HR	REST HR	RUN TYPE	SHOES	NOTES

RUNNING / JOGGING LOG

YEAR _______ MONTH _______

DATE	DISTANCE	TIME	PACE	HR	REST HR	RUN TYPE	SHOES	NOTES

RUNNING / JOGGING LOG

YEAR _______ MONTH _______

DATE	DISTANCE	TIME	PACE	HR	REST HR	RUN TYPE	SHOES	NOTES

RUNNING / JOGGING LOG

YEAR _______ MONTH _______

DATE	DISTANCE	TIME	PACE	HR	REST HR	RUN TYPE	SHOES	NOTES

RUNNING / JOGGING LOG

YEAR _______ MONTH _______

DATE	DISTANCE	TIME	PACE	HR	REST HR	RUN TYPE	SHOES	NOTES

RUNNING / JOGGING LOG

YEAR _______ MONTH _______

DATE	DISTANCE	TIME	PACE	HR	REST HR	RUN TYPE	SHOES	NOTES

RUNNING / JOGGING LOG

YEAR _______ MONTH _______

DATE	DISTANCE	TIME	PACE	HR	REST HR	RUN TYPE	SHOES	NOTES

RUNNING / JOGGING LOG

YEAR _______ MONTH _______

DATE	DISTANCE	TIME	PACE	HR	REST HR	RUN TYPE	SHOES	NOTES

RUNNING / JOGGING LOG

YEAR _______ MONTH _______

DATE	DISTANCE	TIME	PACE	HR	REST HR	RUN TYPE	SHOES	NOTES
DATE	DISTANCE	TIME	PACE	HR	REST HR	RUN TYPE	SHOES	NOTES

RUNNING / JOGGING LOG

YEAR _________ MONTH _________

DATE	DISTANCE	TIME	PACE	HR	REST HR	RUN TYPE	SHOES	NOTES

RUNNING / JOGGING LOG

YEAR _______ MONTH _______

DATE	DISTANCE	TIME	PACE	HR	REST HR	RUN TYPE	SHOES	NOTES

RUNNING / JOGGING LOG

YEAR _________ MONTH _________

DATE	DISTANCE	TIME	PACE	HR	REST HR	RUN TYPE	SHOES	NOTES
DATE	DISTANCE	TIME	PACE	HR	REST HR	RUN TYPE	SHOES	NOTES

RUNNING / JOGGING LOG

YEAR _______ MONTH _______

DATE	DISTANCE	TIME	PACE	HR	REST HR	RUN TYPE	SHOES	NOTES

RUNNING / JOGGING LOG

YEAR _________ MONTH _________

DATE	DISTANCE	TIME	PACE	HR	REST HR	RUN TYPE	SHOES	NOTES

RUNNING / JOGGING LOG

YEAR _______ MONTH _______

DATE	DISTANCE	TIME	PACE	HR	REST HR	RUN TYPE	SHOES	NOTES

RUNNING / JOGGING LOG

YEAR _________ MONTH _________

DATE	DISTANCE	TIME	PACE	HR	REST HR	RUN TYPE	SHOES	NOTES

RUNNING / JOGGING LOG

YEAR _________ MONTH _________

DATE	DISTANCE	TIME	PACE	HR	REST HR	RUN TYPE	SHOES	NOTES

DATE	DISTANCE	TIME	PACE	HR	REST HR	RUN TYPE	SHOES	NOTES

RUNNING / JOGGING LOG

YEAR _______ MONTH _______

DATE	DISTANCE	TIME	PACE	HR	REST HR	RUN TYPE	SHOES	NOTES

RUNNING / JOGGING LOG

YEAR _________ MONTH _________

DATE	DISTANCE	TIME	PACE	HR	REST HR	RUN TYPE	SHOES	NOTES

RUNNING / JOGGING LOG

YEAR ________ MONTH ________

DATE	DISTANCE	TIME	PACE	HR	REST HR	RUN TYPE	SHOES	NOTES

RUNNING / JOGGING LOG

YEAR ______ MONTH ______

DATE	DISTANCE	TIME	PACE	HR	REST HR	RUN TYPE	SHOES	NOTES

RUNNING / JOGGING LOG

YEAR _______ MONTH _______

DATE	DISTANCE	TIME	PACE	HR	REST HR	RUN TYPE	SHOES	NOTES

RUNNING / JOGGING LOG

YEAR _______ MONTH _______

DATE	DISTANCE	TIME	PACE	HR	REST HR	RUN TYPE	SHOES	NOTES

RUNNING / JOGGING LOG

YEAR _________ MONTH _________

DATE	DISTANCE	TIME	PACE	HR	REST HR	RUN TYPE	SHOES	NOTES

RUNNING / JOGGING LOG

YEAR _______ MONTH _______

DATE	DISTANCE	TIME	PACE	HR	REST HR	RUN TYPE	SHOES	NOTES

DATE	DISTANCE	TIME	PACE	HR	REST HR	RUN TYPE	SHOES	NOTES

RUNNING / JOGGING LOG

YEAR _______ MONTH _______

DATE	DISTANCE	TIME	PACE	HR	REST HR	RUN TYPE	SHOES	NOTES

RUNNING / JOGGING LOG

YEAR _______ MONTH _______

DATE	DISTANCE	TIME	PACE	HR	REST HR	RUN TYPE	SHOES	NOTES

RUNNING / JOGGING LOG

YEAR _______ MONTH _______

DATE	DISTANCE	TIME	PACE	HR	REST HR	RUN TYPE	SHOES	NOTES

RUNNING / JOGGING LOG

YEAR _______ MONTH _______

DATE	DISTANCE	TIME	PACE	HR	REST HR	RUN TYPE	SHOES	NOTES

RUNNING / JOGGING LOG

YEAR _______ MONTH _______

DATE	DISTANCE	TIME	PACE	HR	REST HR	RUN TYPE	SHOES	NOTES

RUNNING / JOGGING LOG

YEAR _______ MONTH _______

DATE	DISTANCE	TIME	PACE	HR	REST HR	RUN TYPE	SHOES	NOTES

YEAR _______ MONTH _______

DATE	DISTANCE	TIME	PACE	HR	REST HR	RUN TYPE	SHOES	NOTES

RUNNING / JOGGING LOG

YEAR _______ MONTH _______

DATE	DISTANCE	TIME	PACE	HR	REST HR	RUN TYPE	SHOES	NOTES

RUNNING / JOGGING LOG

YEAR _______ MONTH _______

DATE	DISTANCE	TIME	PACE	HR	REST HR	RUN TYPE	SHOES	NOTES

RUNNING / JOGGING LOG

YEAR _________ MONTH _________

DATE	DISTANCE	TIME	PACE	HR	REST HR	RUN TYPE	SHOES	NOTES

RUNNING / JOGGING LOG

YEAR _______ MONTH _______

DATE	DISTANCE	TIME	PACE	HR	REST HR	RUN TYPE	SHOES	NOTES

RUNNING / JOGGING LOG

YEAR _________ MONTH _________

DATE	DISTANCE	TIME	PACE	HR	REST HR	RUN TYPE	SHOES	NOTES
DATE	DISTANCE	TIME	PACE	HR	REST HR	RUN TYPE	SHOES	NOTES

RUNNING / JOGGING LOG

YEAR _______ MONTH _______

DATE	DISTANCE	TIME	PACE	HR	REST HR	RUN TYPE	SHOES	NOTES
DATE	DISTANCE	TIME	PACE	HR	REST HR	RUN TYPE	SHOES	NOTES

RUNNING / JOGGING LOG

YEAR _______ MONTH _______

DATE	DISTANCE	TIME	PACE	HR	REST HR	RUN TYPE	SHOES	NOTES

DATE	DISTANCE	TIME	PACE	HR	REST HR	RUN TYPE	SHOES	NOTES

RUNNING / JOGGING LOG

YEAR _______ MONTH _______

DATE	DISTANCE	TIME	PACE	HR	REST HR	RUN TYPE	SHOES	NOTES

RUNNING / JOGGING LOG

YEAR _______ MONTH _______

DATE	DISTANCE	TIME	PACE	HR	REST HR	RUN TYPE	SHOES	NOTES

RUNNING / JOGGING LOG

YEAR _______ MONTH _______

DATE	DISTANCE	TIME	PACE	HR	REST HR	RUN TYPE	SHOES	NOTES

RUNNING / JOGGING LOG

YEAR _________ MONTH _________

DATE	DISTANCE	TIME	PACE	HR	REST HR	RUN TYPE	SHOES	NOTES

RUNNING / JOGGING LOG

YEAR _________ MONTH _________

DATE	DISTANCE	TIME	PACE	HR	REST HR	RUN TYPE	SHOES	NOTES
DATE	DISTANCE	TIME	PACE	HR	REST HR	RUN TYPE	SHOES	NOTES

RUNNING / JOGGING LOG

YEAR _______ MONTH _______

DATE	DISTANCE	TIME	PACE	HR	REST HR	RUN TYPE	SHOES	NOTES
DATE	DISTANCE	TIME	PACE	HR	REST HR	RUN TYPE	SHOES	NOTES

RUNNING / JOGGING LOG

YEAR _______ MONTH _______

DATE	DISTANCE	TIME	PACE	HR	REST HR	RUN TYPE	SHOES	NOTES

RUNNING / JOGGING LOG

YEAR _______ MONTH _______

DATE	DISTANCE	TIME	PACE	HR	REST HR	RUN TYPE	SHOES	NOTES

RUNNING / JOGGING LOG

YEAR _________ MONTH _________

DATE	DISTANCE	TIME	PACE	HR	REST HR	RUN TYPE	SHOES	NOTES

DATE	DISTANCE	TIME	PACE	HR	REST HR	RUN TYPE	SHOES	NOTES

RUNNING / JOGGING LOG

YEAR _______ MONTH _______

DATE	DISTANCE	TIME	PACE	HR	REST HR	RUN TYPE	SHOES	NOTES
DATE	DISTANCE	TIME	PACE	HR	REST HR	RUN TYPE	SHOES	NOTES

RUNNING / JOGGING LOG

YEAR _______ MONTH _______

DATE	DISTANCE	TIME	PACE	HR	REST HR	RUN TYPE	SHOES	NOTES

YEAR _______ MONTH _______

DATE	DISTANCE	TIME	PACE	HR	REST HR	RUN TYPE	SHOES	NOTES

RUNNING / JOGGING LOG

YEAR _________ MONTH _________

DATE	DISTANCE	TIME	PACE	HR	REST HR	RUN TYPE	SHOES	NOTES

RUNNING / JOGGING LOG

YEAR _______ MONTH _______

DATE	DISTANCE	TIME	PACE	HR	REST HR	RUN TYPE	SHOES	NOTES

RUNNING / JOGGING LOG

YEAR _______ MONTH _______

DATE	DISTANCE	TIME	PACE	HR	REST HR	RUN TYPE	SHOES	NOTES

RUNNING / JOGGING LOG

YEAR _______ MONTH _______

DATE	DISTANCE	TIME	PACE	HR	REST HR	RUN TYPE	SHOES	NOTES

RUNNING / JOGGING LOG

YEAR _______ MONTH _______

DATE	DISTANCE	TIME	PACE	HR	REST HR	RUN TYPE	SHOES	NOTES
DATE	DISTANCE	TIME	PACE	HR	REST HR	RUN TYPE	SHOES	NOTES

RUNNING / JOGGING LOG

YEAR _______ MONTH _______

DATE	DISTANCE	TIME	PACE	HR	REST HR	RUN TYPE	SHOES		NOTES

RUNNING / JOGGING LOG

YEAR _________ MONTH _________

DATE	DISTANCE	TIME	PACE	HR	REST HR	RUN TYPE	SHOES	NOTES

RUNNING / JOGGING LOG

YEAR _______ MONTH _______

DATE	DISTANCE	TIME	PACE	HR	REST HR	RUN TYPE	SHOES	NOTES

RUNNING / JOGGING LOG

YEAR _______ MONTH _______

DATE	DISTANCE	TIME	PACE	HR	REST HR	RUN TYPE	SHOES	NOTES

RUNNING / JOGGING LOG

YEAR _______ MONTH _______

DATE	DISTANCE	TIME	PACE	HR	REST HR	RUN TYPE	SHOES	NOTES

RUNNING / JOGGING LOG

YEAR _______ MONTH _______

DATE	DISTANCE	TIME	PACE	HR	REST HR	RUN TYPE	SHOES	NOTES

RUNNING / JOGGING LOG

YEAR _________ MONTH _________

DATE	DISTANCE	TIME	PACE	HR	REST HR	RUN TYPE	SHOES	NOTES

RUNNING / JOGGING LOG

YEAR _______ MONTH _______

DATE	DISTANCE	TIME	PACE	HR	REST HR	RUN TYPE	SHOES	NOTES

RUNNING / JOGGING LOG

YEAR _________ MONTH _________

DATE	DISTANCE	TIME	PACE	HR	REST HR	RUN TYPE	SHOES	NOTES

RUNNING / JOGGING LOG

YEAR _________ MONTH _________

DATE	DISTANCE	TIME	PACE	HR	REST HR	RUN TYPE	SHOES	NOTES

RUNNING / JOGGING LOG

YEAR _______ MONTH _______

DATE	DISTANCE	TIME	PACE	HR	REST HR	RUN TYPE	SHOES	NOTES

RUNNING / JOGGING LOG

YEAR _______ MONTH _______

DATE	DISTANCE	TIME	PACE	HR	REST HR	RUN TYPE	SHOES	NOTES
DATE	DISTANCE	TIME	PACE	HR	REST HR	RUN TYPE	SHOES	NOTES

RUNNING / JOGGING LOG

YEAR _______ MONTH _______

DATE	DISTANCE	TIME	PACE	HR	REST HR	RUN TYPE	SHOES	NOTES

RUNNING / JOGGING LOG

YEAR _______ MONTH _______

DATE	DISTANCE	TIME	PACE	HR	REST HR	RUN TYPE	SHOES	NOTES

RUNNING / JOGGING LOG

YEAR _______ MONTH _______

DATE	DISTANCE	TIME	PACE	HR	REST HR	RUN TYPE	SHOES	NOTES
DATE	DISTANCE	TIME	PACE	HR	REST HR	RUN TYPE	SHOES	NOTES

RUNNING / JOGGING LOG

YEAR _________ MONTH _________

DATE	DISTANCE	TIME	PACE	HR	REST HR	RUN TYPE	SHOES	NOTES

RUNNING / JOGGING LOG

YEAR _________ MONTH _________

DATE	DISTANCE	TIME	PACE	HR	REST HR	RUN TYPE	SHOES	NOTES
DATE	DISTANCE	TIME	PACE	HR	REST HR	RUN TYPE	SHOES	NOTES

RUNNING / JOGGING LOG

YEAR _______ MONTH _______

DATE	DISTANCE	TIME	PACE	HR	REST HR	RUN TYPE	SHOES	NOTES

RUNNING / JOGGING LOG

YEAR _________ MONTH _________

DATE	DISTANCE	TIME	PACE	HR	REST HR	RUN TYPE	SHOES	NOTES

RUNNING / JOGGING LOG

YEAR _______ MONTH _______

DATE	DISTANCE	TIME	PACE	HR	REST HR	RUN TYPE	SHOES	NOTES

RUNNING / JOGGING LOG

YEAR _________ MONTH _________

DATE	DISTANCE	TIME	PACE	HR	REST HR	RUN TYPE	SHOES	NOTES

RUNNING / JOGGING LOG

YEAR _______ MONTH _______

DATE	DISTANCE	TIME	PACE	HR	REST HR	RUN TYPE	SHOES	NOTES

RUNNING / JOGGING LOG

YEAR _______ MONTH _______

DATE	DISTANCE	TIME	PACE	HR	REST HR	RUN TYPE	SHOES	NOTES
DATE	DISTANCE	TIME	PACE	HR	REST HR	RUN TYPE	SHOES	NOTES

RUNNING / JOGGING LOG

YEAR _______ MONTH _______

DATE	DISTANCE	TIME	PACE	HR	REST HR	RUN TYPE	SHOES	NOTES

RUNNING / JOGGING LOG

YEAR _______ MONTH _______

DATE	DISTANCE	TIME	PACE	HR	REST HR	RUN TYPE	SHOES	NOTES

RUNNING / JOGGING LOG

YEAR _________ MONTH _________

DATE	DISTANCE	TIME	PACE	HR	REST HR	RUN TYPE	SHOES	NOTES

RUNNING / JOGGING LOG

YEAR _______ MONTH _______

DATE	DISTANCE	TIME	PACE	HR	REST HR	RUN TYPE	SHOES	NOTES
DATE	DISTANCE	TIME	PACE	HR	REST HR	RUN TYPE	SHOES	NOTES

RUNNING / JOGGING LOG

YEAR _________ MONTH _________

DATE	DISTANCE	TIME	PACE	HR	REST HR	RUN TYPE	SHOES	NOTES

RUNNING / JOGGING LOG

YEAR ______ MONTH ______

DATE	DISTANCE	TIME	PACE	HR	REST HR	RUN TYPE	SHOES	NOTES

RUNNING / JOGGING LOG

YEAR _________ MONTH _________

DATE	DISTANCE	TIME	PACE	HR	REST HR	RUN TYPE	SHOES	NOTES

RUNNING / JOGGING LOG

YEAR _______ MONTH _______

DATE	DISTANCE	TIME	PACE	HR	REST HR	RUN TYPE	SHOES	NOTES

RUNNING / JOGGING LOG

YEAR ______ MONTH ______

DATE	DISTANCE	TIME	PACE	HR	REST HR	RUN TYPE	SHOES	NOTES

RUNNING / JOGGING LOG

YEAR _______ MONTH _______

DATE	DISTANCE	TIME	PACE	HR	REST HR	RUN TYPE	SHOES	NOTES

RUNNING / JOGGING LOG

YEAR _______ MONTH _______

DATE	DISTANCE	TIME	PACE	HR	REST HR	RUN TYPE	SHOES	NOTES

RUNNING / JOGGING LOG

YEAR _______ MONTH _______

DATE	DISTANCE	TIME	PACE	HR	REST HR	RUN TYPE	SHOES	NOTES

RUNNING / JOGGING LOG

YEAR _______ MONTH _______

DATE	DISTANCE	TIME	PACE	HR	REST HR	RUN TYPE	SHOES	NOTES

RUNNING / JOGGING LOG

YEAR ______ MONTH ______

DATE	DISTANCE	TIME	PACE	HR	REST HR	RUN TYPE	SHOES	NOTES

RUNNING / JOGGING LOG

YEAR ______ MONTH ______

DATE	DISTANCE	TIME	PACE	HR	REST HR	RUN TYPE	SHOES	NOTES

RUNNING / JOGGING LOG

YEAR _______ MONTH _______

DATE	DISTANCE	TIME	PACE	HR	REST HR	RUN TYPE	SHOES	NOTES

RUNNING / JOGGING LOG

YEAR _______ MONTH _______

DATE	DISTANCE	TIME	PACE	HR	REST HR	RUN TYPE	SHOES	NOTES

RUNNING / JOGGING LOG

YEAR _______ MONTH _______

DATE	DISTANCE	TIME	PACE	HR	REST HR	RUN TYPE	SHOES	NOTES
DATE	DISTANCE	TIME	PACE	HR	REST HR	RUN TYPE	SHOES	NOTES